DATE DUE

AUG 1 4 2007	

DEMCO, INC. 38-2931

SURFING
RULES, TIPS, STRATEGY, AND SAFETY

NAIMA GREEN

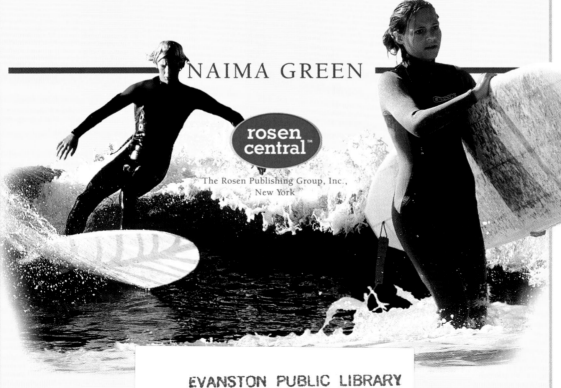

rosen
central™

The Rosen Publishing Group, Inc.,
New York

To Birdie

Published in 2005 by The Rosen Publishing Group, Inc.
29 East 21st Street, New York, NY 10010

Copyright © 2005 by The Rosen Publishing Group, Inc.

First Edition

Library of Congress Cataloging-in-Publication Data

Green, Naima.
Surfing: rules, tips, strategy, and safety / by Naima Green.—1st ed.
    p. cm.—(Sports from coast to coast)
Includes bibliographical references and index.
ISBN 1-4042-0184-X (library binding)
1. Surfing—Juvenile literature.
I. Title. II. Series.
GV840.S8G73 2005
797.3'2—dc22

                                                          2004000295

Manufactured in the United States of America

CONTENTS

Chapter One   History of Surfing   4

Chapter Two   Getting Started   10

Chapter Three   Diving In   20

Chapter Four   Surfing Today   32

Glossary   42

For More Information   43

For Further Reading   44

Bibliography   45

Index   46

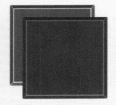
History of Surfing

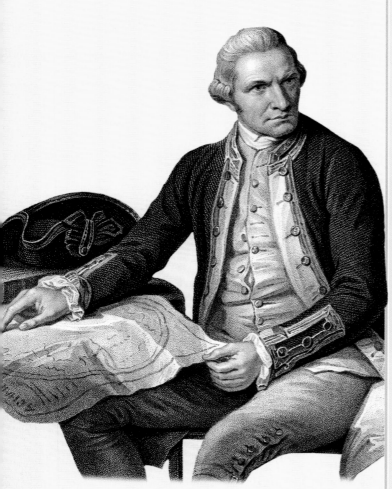

Legendary navigator Captain James Cook was the first European to visit the Hawaiian Islands. He originally named them the Sandwich Islands, after his friend the Earl of Sandwich.

The year was 1778. English sea captain James Cook stood at the bow of his mighty ship, the *Resolution*, while his men surrounded him, looking ahead to their unknown destination. As they sailed toward the islands of Hawaii, Cook's sailors stood in awe, staring at the lush land before them. Steep volcanic cliffs barreled down to the black sand beaches of Kealakekua Bay, the place the Hawaiians call the Pathway of the Gods. As the ship sailed into shallower water, the crew saw brightly colored fish, dashing this way and that throughout the undersea jungle of coral and seaweed. The men saw things they had never imagined. They might have thought they had found the most beautiful place on Earth.

As they approached the shore, men aboard Cook's ship strained their eyes to glimpse the native peoples who gathered along the Hawaiian coast. The men aboard the ship looked to the surrounding ocean for those who might greet them. There were no boats, however, that met Cook's crew in the surf. Instead, it was a Hawaiian kneeling on a long wooden board and gracefully skimming the waves as he approached Cook's ship. This would be the first time the Western world would see this art form of surfing that is a complete union of nature and sport.

When we think of surfing, what often comes to mind is a group of tanned beach boys with brightly colored boards, sliding gracefully along the tips of foamy waves of untouched white sand beaches. Surfing, however, has very different origins. Surfing was a traditional practice of the indigenous people of Hawaii. Although many of us think of Hawaii as part of the United States, it did not become the fiftieth state until 1959 and was actually an independent nation until 1893. But no matter the changes, Hawaii's surfing traditions remained. Surfing has long been practiced on the paradise islands of Hawaii and has remained an important part of Hawaiian culture.

The Birthplace of Surfing

Around the fourth century, groups of people from the South Pacific islands of Polynesia traveled the ocean, discovering previously unknown islands. Ancient folklore indicates that the islands of Hawaii were discovered by a Polynesian fisherman named Hawai-iloa, who got lost on a long fishing trip. Soon afterward, when other Polynesian travelers got word of the beautiful, untouched islands of Hawaii, many settlers would make their way there.

The Polynesians en route to Hawaii were mostly from the small islands of Fiji, Tonga, and Samoa. They were accustomed to traveling thousands of miles in canoes, which were built out of hollowed trees. They used objects found in nature as their tools for shaping the canoes: stones or bones, for example.

Once a boat was constructed, the hardest part was yet to come: traveling some 2,000 miles across the massive ocean all the way to Hawaii. For navigation, the Polynesians carefully read the clues and signs offered by nature, such as the movement of the wind, the flights of seabirds, and the stars at night. Those who could endure the long trip would become the original settlers of the Hawaiian Islands, which historians believe was settled by the fourth century AD.

It is not surprising that a group of people who found their home in Hawaii by traveling the wide ocean would have such a deep connection to it. Not only did the ocean lead them to their new home, but it also sustained the people with its vast natural resources. For islanders like the Hawaiians, the ocean is the vein that pumps life, food, water, and faith into the heart of the culture. Just as the Inuit have many words for ice and snow, the people of Hawaii have just as many words for water or ocean. It is even believed that the children of ancient Hawaiians learned to swim before they learned to walk!

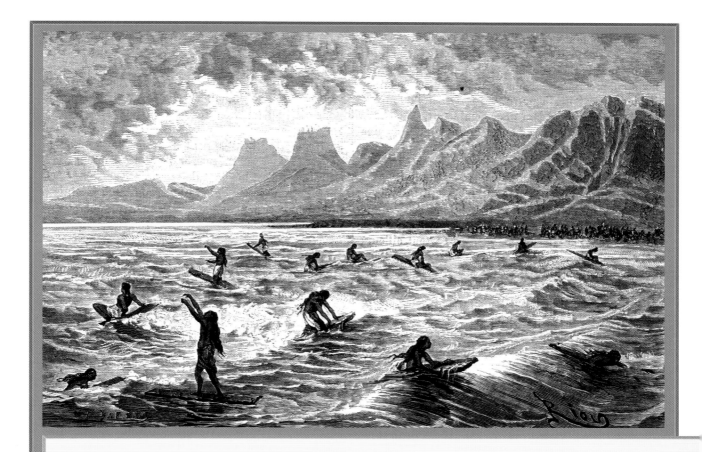

Ancient Hawaiians called board surfing *he`e nalu,* which means "wave sliding." It was often performed by kneeling or laying on the board. Hawaiians also developed body surfing, called *kaha nalu*, which was then performed without a board.

The ocean, however, was not something the people relied on only for necessities like travel, nourishment, and religious inspiration. It was also a place the Hawaiians could look to for fun, and often, fun came in the form of surfing, canoeing, and other water sports.

Surfing was actually a sport practiced by people from all walks of life in ancient Hawaii. Not only did the Hawaiian teenagers practice surfing, so did Hawaiian royalty. According to historians, Hawaiian kings and queens would show off their skill and power through surfing! A

The Duke

During the early twentieth century, when surfing was still relatively unknown to most Americans, surfing clubs began popping up around Hawaiian beaches. Once the clubs were established, people began to take notice of the sport. Soon, surfing stars were born. One of those budding beach celebrities was named Duke Paoa Kahanamoku, or "the Duke." He was founder of the Hui Nalu Club on the Big Island of Hawaii.

The Duke first became famous as an Olympic champion in freestyle swimming. More than a surfer, the Duke went on to start his own surf team, market a whole line of surf products, open a nightclub, and even star in Hollywood movies. The Duke was a busy man, and he used his worldwide influence to promote his most beloved pastime—surfing!

The Duke even inspired a classic surfing competition in Hawaii that became legendary during the 1960s and 1970s. Called the Duke Classic, this annual competition is held in honor of the sport's first living legend.

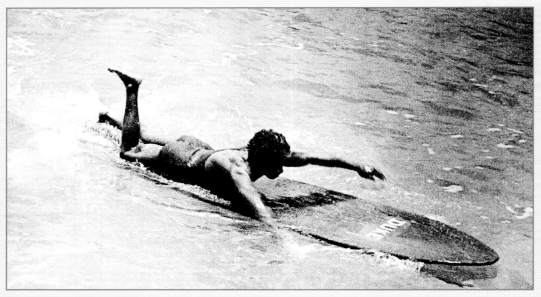

The Duke, also known as the Big Kahuna, made his own surfboards using the techniques of ancient Hawaiians. His board was made from a koa tree. It was 16 feet long and weighed 114 pounds.

king or queen was expected to be an extremely skilled surfer. If he or she had a big wipeout in front of the community, it would be very embarrassing and sometimes even damaging to his or her popularity.

There were special boards only members of royalty were allowed to ride. These boards often measured up to twenty-four feet long! The boards used by common people were only about half that length. Hawaiian royalty even had designated beaches where they surfed. If a commoner set foot on that beach, he or she would have to face the consequences of trespassing on royal land.

By the time Captain Cook arrived from Europe, Hawaiians had been settled for generations. It was not until 1779, during a return trip to the Polynesian Islands, that Cook encountered surfers standing on their boards in Hawaii. He and his crew were captivated— they had never seen something so unique as people riding waves on a piece of wood!

Later, there would be countless other Europeans to come. Many of them were missionaries out to convert the native peoples to Christianity. After the arrival of the Europeans, however, the surfing culture would begin its decline, mainly because of new restrictions placed on the Hawaiians by the missionaries. For a long time after the Christians arrived in Hawaii, surfing was strictly banned. Surfing would have almost disappeared if it were not for a few Hawaiians who surfed in secret, resisting the new rules imposed on them.

By the mid-nineteenth century, Hawaiians began to break away from the strict rules placed on them by the Christian world. They knew that surfing was not a bad activity but an important and fun part of their culture. As the practice of surfing reemerged, people took notice.

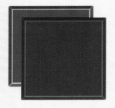

CHAPTER TWO

Getting Started

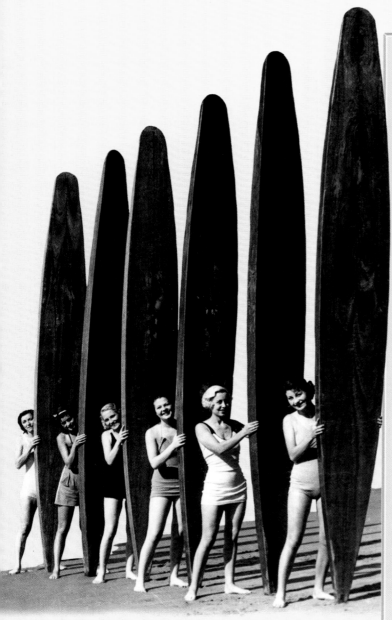

Before the 1960s, enormous wooden surfboards, called longboards, were commonly used. Today's surfboard is much smaller and lighter.

One of the greatest things about the sport of surfing is that you need only three basic things: your body, a surfboard, and a wave. Also, it is possible to practice this solitary sport with just one or two people, instead of with an entire team. The surfer sets his or her own schedule, and only the waves influence whether you go surfing or not!

Evolution of the Board

In the days of Captain Cook, surfboards were heavy and hard to handle. This is because they were made of hard woods found in the forests, unlike the light, fiberglass surfboards used today. Also, the ancient surfboards were a lot longer, requiring much more strength to haul them through the sand and into the ocean. Plus, when the board got away from a surfer, he or she had a harder time bringing it back into the surf.

At the turn of the twentieth century, however, surfboards were being made of different materials—materials that were lighter and stronger than wood found in the Hawaiian forests. Surfboard shapers, the people who make surfboards, began using lighter woods, such as balsa or plywood. These new, lighter boards were much easier to transport through the long stretches of sand that lay before the waves. These boards were also much easier to handle in the ocean.

Beginning in the early 1960s, when surfing's popularity exploded, traditional boards began to change shape radically. Since then, contemporary surfboards have become shorter and shorter. In the late 1960s, the introduction of fiberglass changed the face of surfing. Fiberglass is even lighter and more buoyant than the lightest wood used to make surfboards. Not only are fiberglass boards easier to carry around, they also allow their owners to perform more advanced maneuvers in the water.

The Big Guns: The Longboard

Before the 1960s, longboards, or surfboards which measured about nine feet or more, were the most common. Longboards were the traditional "big guns" of Hawaii. They allowed surfers to ride huge waves, like those found on the north shore of the Hawaiian island of Oahu.

Surfing changed when shorter boards—around six feet long—hit the scene by the 1960s, and surfers realized how much more mobility they had on them. The boards just kept getting shorter and shorter as surfers realized they could do more stunts and specialty moves with them.

For decades it seemed as though the longboard had vanished from the horizon. However, in recent years some young surfers brought back the use of the longboard. They started using them as an homage to the ancient Hawaiians, to experience surfing the way it had been before the sport hit the mainstream. These purists attempted surfing with ultralong wooden boards, and with no leashes or special equipment. Although longboard surfers may not be able to perform lots of stunts on these boards, they can achieve much more grace, and sometimes, an even longer ride.

Today's Surfboards

If you walk into a surf shop these days, you will see a few choices of surfboards. You'll need to spend time making your decision and always ask lots of questions! This will ensure that you'll find the right board to meet your needs. Here are the basics on what to look for:

Soft Boards

These foam boards are the lightest, yet most durable kind of surfboard. They are also the easiest to handle in the water. Because of their durability, soft boards are the best kind of board for the beginning surfer. They can endure wipeout after wipeout—something the beginner will spend a lot of time doing!

Surfing the Longboard

When surfing on a longboard, skill is determined through style. This is the way the surfer handles the board in the water. Since there is more surface area, or space to move around on the long board, the surfer must take little steps across it during his or her ride. These small, quick steps are to keep the surfer balanced. From the beach, these quick steps look more like a graceful, stylish dance. The uniqueness of this "dance," and the grace with which it is performed, determine the surfer's style. Doing this dance on a short surfboard would be impossible. Today, some competitions are broken down into two categories, longboard and shortboard.

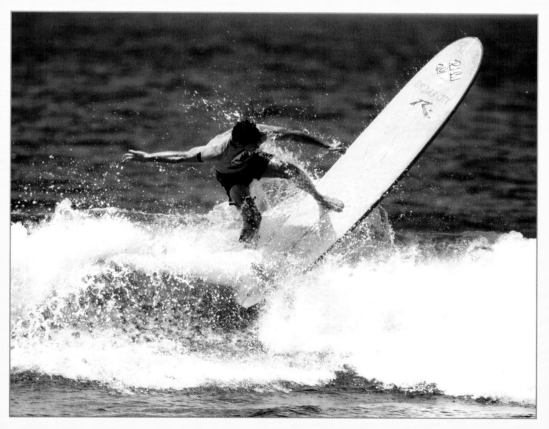

Longboards allow a surfer to maneuver around small waves. To maintain balance on these waves, a surfer will put his or her "toes on the nose" or "hang ten" toes off the nose of the board.

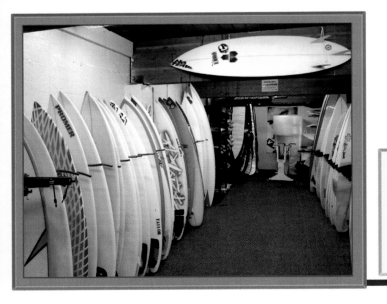

When buying a board, it's a good idea to ask the surf shop salesperson plenty of questions about which board will be right for you. Also, make sure that the board is in perfect condition and has no scratches or dings.

Molded Surfboards

Molded surfboards are made of two sections of fiberglass molded together with a polyurethane (a specific kind of plastic) center. These boards are not as light as the soft boards, yet not as breakable as the custom boards. Molded surfboards are the most popular with surfers with intermediate experience levels.

Custom Boards

Custom boards are another type of light surfboard. As the name implies, these boards can be made specifically for the individual surfer. Surfboard shapers can customize everything about the board, including color, design, and even what kind of wave it should perform best on. However, these are the most breakable boards, as well as the most expensive. For these reasons alone, the beginning surfer should leave custom boards to expert surfers.

The Fin

Some surfers prefer boards with fins, or rudders, that are connected to the bottom of the board, giving the surfer better control. For years since

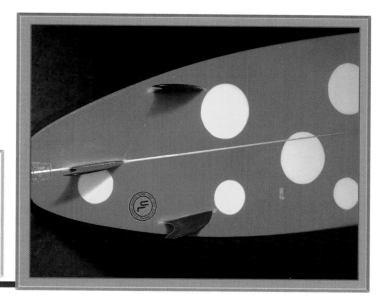

The triple-fin board made surfing a little less difficult for surfers. Today, some boards come with detachable fins that can be removed or placed in the opposite direction.

the dawn of surfing, only one fin was used on the board. However, the development of twin fins during the 1970s was important in the evolution of the surfboard. Twin fins allowed the surfer much more control over his or her board. This also helped the surfer gain better mobility when surfing the smaller waves found in shallower waters.

In 1981, surfer Simon Anderson took fin changes even further with the introduction of the triple-fin surfboard. On that first three-fin board, Anderson won the prestigious Bells Beach Contest and became an international surfing celebrity.

Accessories for the Surfboard

Although the surfer's main tool is his or her board, many choose different accessories to help them along the way. Although these accessories are not always a must, they can make surfing much more comfortable and enjoyable, especially for the novice.

Wax

Surfing wax is used to give the surfer traction on the board, or a surface to grip, so he or she does not slip while standing on the board. Wax is rubbed into the face, or top side of the board. Sometimes sand is applied

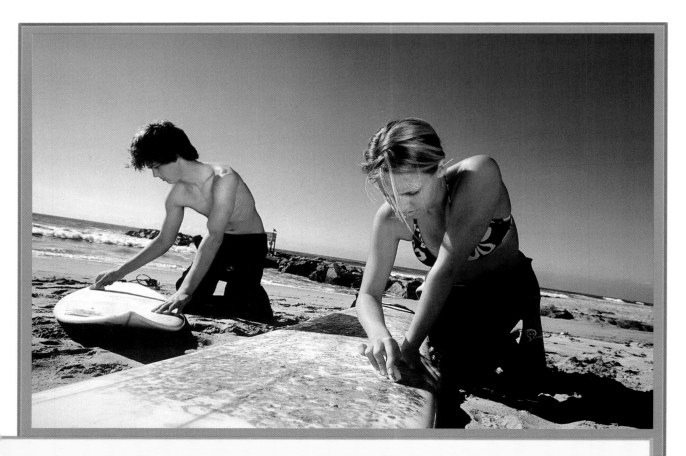

Reapplying wax to a board can waste valuable surfing time! Instead of using board wax, some surfers use expensive but time-saving deck grips. Deck grips are permanent board adhesives that give the surfer better traction on the board.

to the mixture to give the board even more traction. After all, it would be pretty embarrassing to slip off a board after catching the perfect wave! Before buying wax, be sure to ask an experienced surfer which kind to buy because there are different types for various water temperatures.

Leash

Even though old-time surfers never used this accessory for their surfboards, the invention of the leash has saved many a lost board!

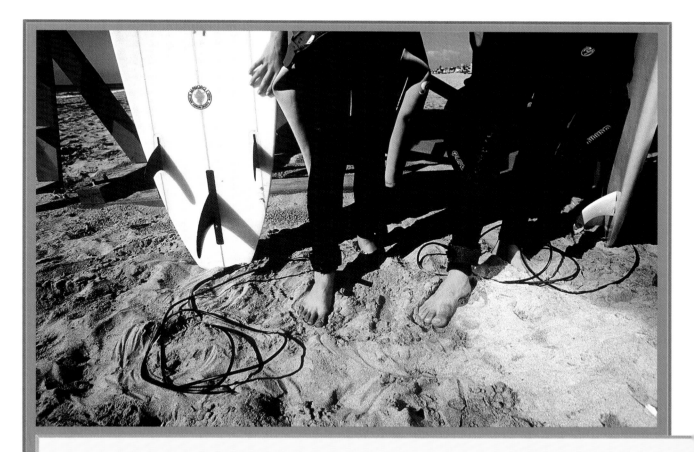

Using a leash not only saves your board, it can also save you a long, tiresome swim back to the beach. When selling a surfboard, retailers will usually include a free leash. They know it isn't fun to lose the board you just paid good money for!

By simply wrapping a Velcro strip around your ankle and connecting it to your board, you can be sure of retrieving your board after a wipeout.

Noseguards

Some surfers choose to protect the nose, or tip, of their surfboard with these rubber guards. This way, scratches and nicks from the ocean floor or coral reefs won't ruin your board. Sometimes, tiny cracks can

Surfing Without a Surfboard: Skim Boards and Boogie Boards

Skim boards are rounded plywood or fiberglass boards that are used to slide across the sand at the base of the shore, where there is only a very thin layer of water. This activity is popular with kids, partly because the boards are fairly inexpensive. As the wave is either coming in or going back out to sea (when the depth of the water is only a couple of inches), the skimboard is thrown onto the shore and surfed until there is no water left to ride.

Boogie boards are foam boards that are much wider than surfboards, but much shorter. Instead of standing up for the ride, the boogie boarder rides waves on his or her belly. That means it takes a lot less energy to ride a great wave! Although the boogie boarder could never ride the big waves of Oahu's North Shore, the board performs excellently on small to medium waves.

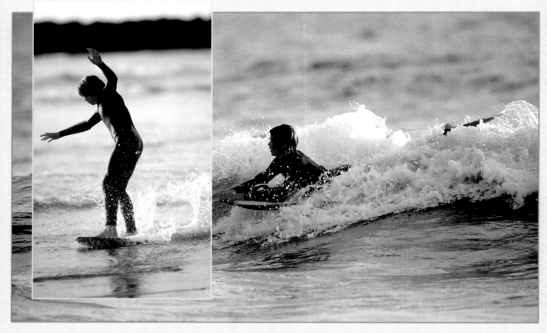

Riding a skim board (*left*) or a boogie board (*right*) is often viewed as an easier form of surfing. However, many of these boarders add complex gymnastic moves and techniques when riding a wave.

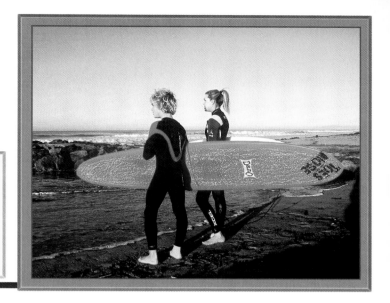

Wet suits allow a tiny bit of water to come between the skin and the suit. Body heat then warms the water, which is insulated by a neoprene layer in the wet suit.

turn into bigger ones, so this accessory is very handy for prolonging the life of a surfboard.

Wet Suits

Wet suits are body coverings with linings, made so that a surfer can stay in the water for hour after hour without getting cold. Just as marine mammals such as whales and dolphins have an extra layer to protect them from the cold, so should the surfer. Wet suits also protect against scrapes and cuts from the ocean floor. There are different wet suits for colder and warmer waters, so be sure to ask someone experienced for advice before buying one.

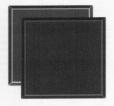

CHAPTER THREE

Diving In

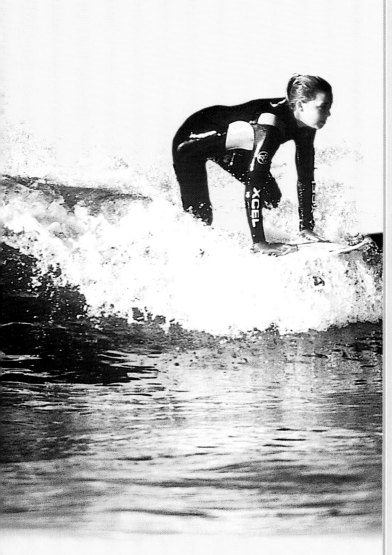

Once you've learned how to pop up, you're almost there! Popping up can be the most difficult technique to master for novice surfers.

Even though the beginning surfer may want to rush into the water as soon as he or she catches sight of the beach, it is necessary to have patience. It is very important to learn exactly how to approach the surf, and what to do once you're in it. There are some technical moves to learn on the beach before even getting one toe wet. Even though this book will help the beginning surfer learn about the sport, a helpful and patient teacher is highly recommended.

The Popup

Every beginning surfer needs to try his or her hand at the popup maneuver. Starting out crouched in the sand, the novice should try to jump onto his or her board, and into the stance of a surfer. "Belly to feet" is another way to describe the popup, and it must be performed in one quick fluid motion.

To decide which side of the board to start from, figure out which foot feels best in front. Usually, people tend to know instinctively which way feels natural, but sometimes it is necessary to try the popup on both sides before making a decision. If the left foot is forward, it is in the regular, or most common stance (just like being right-handed). If the right foot is forward, the stance is called goofy-foot. This is not an insulting nickname, it's just the basic term used to describe lefties in the world of surfing.

Basically, performing the beach popup is practice for exactly what is required in the ocean. Many beginning surfers practice the popup hundreds of times before actually diving in.

Getting Wet

Before stepping into the ocean, the surfer first makes sure all his or her accessories are being properly held. This means carrying the leash in one hand and having it neatly wound around the board for safety. Otherwise, the surfer could trip and fall and experience a wipeout before even getting near the water! Also, the board must be carried in a specific way. If there are fins on it, the fins should face in, toward the surfer, who should walk into the ocean with the nose, or tip, facing forward.

Duckdiving

Before actually paddling out to the big waves, it is important to try out more maneuvers in order to be completely prepared. Sometimes it is best to try out these moves in shallow water first.

As the surfer paddles out into deeper water, he or she comes upon white water, the foamy area of the surf created after a wave crashes. To bypass the white water without getting toppled over, it is necessary to learn a move called the duckdive.

Duckdiving is performed by ducking your head under the waves that are about to crash above you. This is to avoid any impact with oncoming waves. The goal of the successful duckdive is to imitate the ducks or seabirds that look for food underwater. Usually with one knee propped on the board, the surfer dunks his or her head under the water just behind the front of the board, with his or her head tucked under the neck area, like a duck. Once under the water, the board's buoyancy causes the board to shoot up toward the surface again, safely past the waves. The surfer continues doing this maneuver until he or she paddles out past the white water.

Looking for the Lineup

Once the surfer is well past the white water and has had plenty of practice on both the beach and the smaller waves, it is time to look for the "lineup." As the surfer paddles out into deeper and deeper

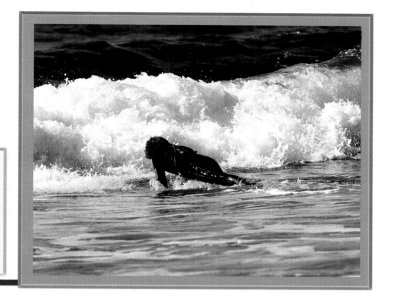

A brave surfer paddles out to the white water, ready to duckdive beneath the crest. As she approaches the white water, she paddles to gather as much speed as possible.

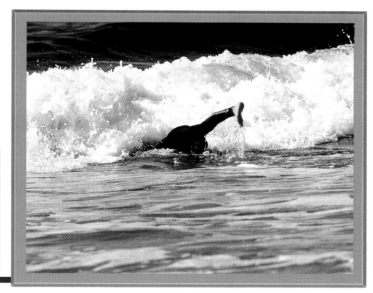

Next, the surfer begins to duck under the wave. She pushes herself downward at an angle by kicking up her strongest leg, while leaving the other leg bent on the board.

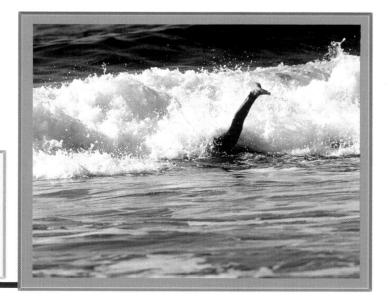

Mission accomplished! The surfer has successfully ducked beneath the wave and will now point the nose of her board to float herself toward the water's surface.

water, he or she will notice a line of other surfers, all waiting for the perfect wave. Just like in everyday life, when waiting in line it is considered rude to jump in front of the person ahead of you. The same rule of thumb applies in surfing. The beginning surfer may learn the hard way if he or she attempts skipping another surfer in the lineup. What would happen if you jump in front of the line at a grocery store?

Once in the lineup, the surfer must look for many things in order to catch the perfect wave. The best way to achieve this is by watching other surfers and paying attention to the kinds of waves they ride. Watch for the waves that create successful rides, and for the waves that wipe out surfers. As with any sport, learning how to surf takes time, patience, and the willingness to ask for advice when in doubt.

Catching the Perfect Wave

The surfer must catch the wave just as it is beginning to break. At the same time, he or she should try to steady himself or herself on the board and attempt a popup, just like beginners practice on the beach. In one quick motion, the surfer should move smoothly from the water to the board, or belly to board. Many beginners get discouraged after their first attempts at standing on the board, but it is necessary to try again and again. It sometimes takes beginners several practice waves before being able to stand successfully on a surfboard.

This surfer, thinking he has found the perfect wave, attempts to barrel under the wave's curl. From December to February, Hawaii is a good place to look for the perfect wave. Some Hawaiian waves reach several stories high!

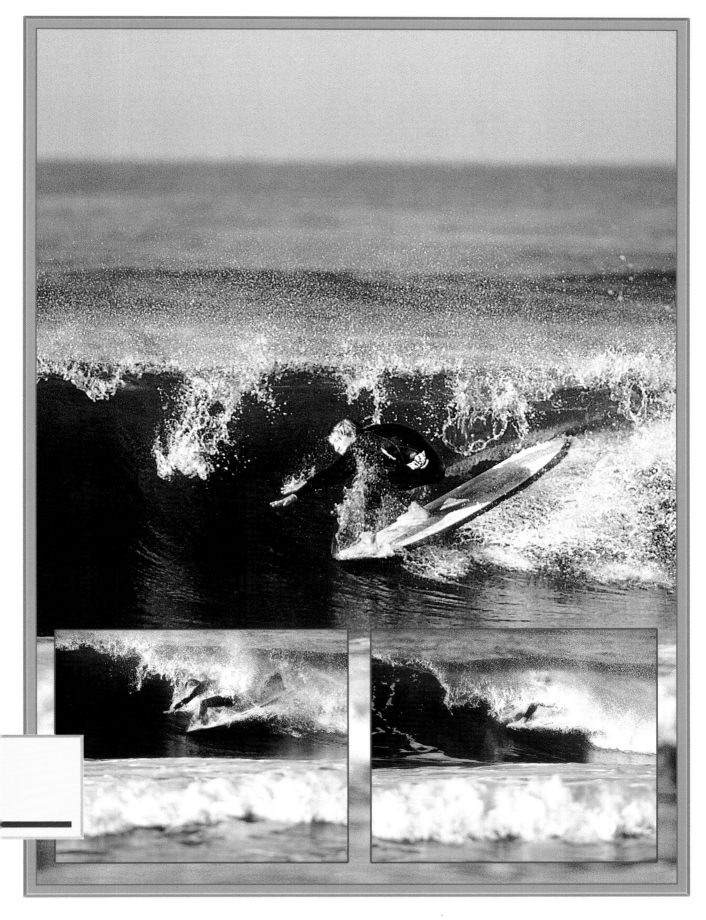

When preparing for a day of surfing, the novice should always follow the clues he or she receives from nature to determine the surf. It is important to remember that the best surfers see the ocean as something they must combine themselves with, not fight against. That said, he or she must remember that it takes perfect harmony of the ocean and the surfer to achieve the best ride possible.

The best surfers hit the beach really early, sometimes before the sun even rises. These early hours are said to hold the best waves because the waves are at their highest because of the high tide at that hour. Take it from the pros and go out early!

Surfing Etiquette

The beginning surfer must be aware of a few rules of etiquette, including being respectful to other surfers, when successfully navigating the waves. These rules can also help the surfer make friends and gain respect in the lineup.

Right of Way

Just as in driving, one of surfing's most important rules is the right of way. The first surfer on a particular wave, or the surfer who is closest to the curl of the wave, has the right of way. The curl is the part of the wave that creates a tunnel when it is just about to break. This basically means that if someone is already riding a wave, get out of the way.

Always Help Other Surfers in Trouble

If you cannot paddle out to help a surfer in distress, be sure to call out to other surfers in the surrounding area. This is one of the most

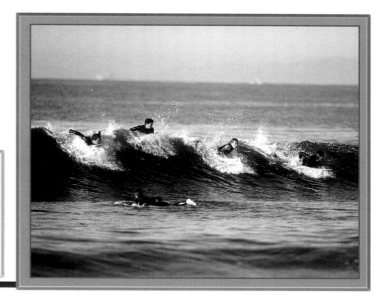

The first person to reach the curl will sometimes shout, "I got it!" or, "Coming down!" to warn nearby surfers to get out of the way.

important rules in surfing. Everyone must be willing to drop even the most perfect wave to help a fellow surfer in need.

Hold On

Never let go of the surfboard, especially around crowds or other surfers. This is mainly because the board could hurt someone, plus, you could lose your precious surfboard.

Avoid Hostility

The lineup can be a very competitive place, and new surfers are often picked on a little. If any surfer seems overly aggressive, just avoid him or her. There is never any need to fight or argue, especially over a wave.

Only Surf Waves You Can Handle

Know your limitations. In other words, a beginner surfer shouldn't expect to paddle out and surf the biggest wave around. Leave the big waves to the pros, because if you don't, you'll probably get hurt. The ocean can wield overwhelming power, and you can find yourself at the mercy of these big waves. This rule also helps with overcrowding, as it

Sharks and Surfing

Of all words in the English language, the word "shark" probably evokes the most fear for surfers! Sharks are among the most feared creatures in the ocean, and possibly in the world. Some spiritual surfers see the shark as their protector, but many contemporary surfers see sharks as their strongest adversaries in the ocean.

Different nicknames exist for different sharks, depending on a surfer's geographic location. For instance, in Australia, the shark most commonly linked to shark attacks is the infamous great white, or the "man in the grey suit." In tropical areas where the water is warm, tiger sharks, or "terries," are mainly responsible for shark attacks. However, shark attacks are extremely rare.

The most important thing to remember is this: Humans are not part of a shark's natural diet. If a shark attacks, it is only because the shark thinks the surfer or swimmer is a seal, an otter, or another marine mammal. Like any wild animal, the shark is probably more afraid of you than you are of it. Before going surfing for the first time, consider doing a bit of research on sharks. Find out which ones are in your particular surf area, and follow instructions on what to do and wear so you don't attract them.

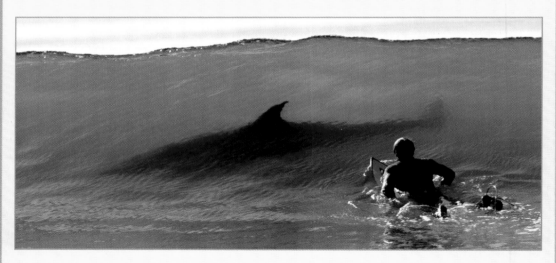

Shark! Actually, it's a dolphin. A surfer in California is relieved to find out that a suspicious-looking fin belongs to a friendly dolphin rather than to a hungry shark. As a surfer, it is always important to be on your guard. Shark attacks are extremely rare, but it is always good to be alert.

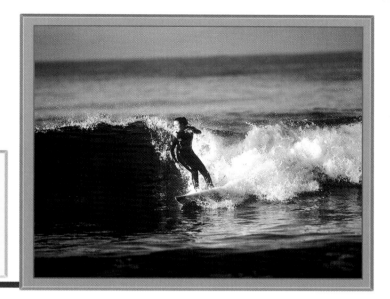

The lineup can be confusing for a new surfer. It's important to apologize if you make a mistake. Even the best surfers will remember what it was like to be a beginner.

instructs the inexperienced surfer to free up lineup space for waves he or she cannot yet surf.

Never "Drop In" on Anyone

Never dropping in on another surfer means never charging a wave that someone else is already riding. Dropping in can lead to collisions between surfers and cause serious injuries. "Snaking" someone is just as bad. Dropping in usually differs from snaking in one way: Snakers come in from the side and whip in front of another surfer, whereas in dropping in, the surfer steals the wave from behind.

Safety First

Sometimes it is easy to become carried away by the excitement and beauty of the ocean and the surf. But it is important to understand that safety comes first. Do not take any unnecessary risks. Wait to attempt the big waves until you are an experienced and well-traveled surfer.

Never, Ever Surf Alone

Although the tranquility of the ocean at first light would seem like something to experience alone, always take a friend along. The ocean

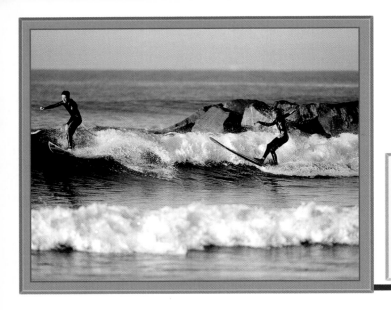

Two surfing buddies share a small wave. Surfing with a friend is not only a safe way to surf but can produce life-long friendships.

is powerful and unpredictable. You could drown, you could run into trouble with dangerous sea animals, or you could get caught up in a reef too deeply. A friend should be surfing with you at all times to help you out in case of an emergency and vice versa.

Watch the Ocean for at Least Thirty Minutes Before Paddling Out

When paddling out to the lineup, pay close attention to the face of the ocean. Look for abnormalities in the surface, which might indicate the presence of rocks, reefs, or shallow water.

Always Wear Sunscreen

Exposure to the sun can be dangerous, especially since the sun's rays are actually magnified by the surface of the water. Always wear a waterproof sunscreen with an SPF of at least 30 when surfing.

Be Aware of Riptides or Currents

Strong, pounding waves are not the only thing to watch out for in the ocean. Riptides are strong currents in the ocean that can pull a surfer

Surfing Lingo

The world of surfing has its own lingo of sorts. If the beginning surfer studies up on these words and phrases, he or she might make an impression in the lineup!

Bone crusher: A big wave that breaks with extreme force.

Buoy: Someone who floats around, never takes a wave, and is often in the way.

Carving up the mob: Australian term for a reckless ride as one surfer cuts through a group of surfers or swimmers.

Casper: A nickname for a tourist or newcomer who has yet to get a tan—named after the famous friendly cartoon ghost.

Stickbug stance: Riding a longboard, squatting with your feet spread wide apart and your butt sticking out.

Tubular: Valleyspeak for "cool," as in "totally tubular."

Walking the dog: Walking forward and backward on a surfboard to alter speed.

or swimmer out to sea. If caught in a riptide, the surfer must paddle or swim parallel to the shore until the current subsides, then swim back to shore. Do not swim straight back toward the beach. Do not swim directly against the current. Swim in the direction that offers the least resistance, and remember, you can't see riptides and deadly currents, but they are there—always!

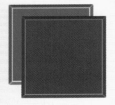

CHAPTER FOUR

Surfing Today

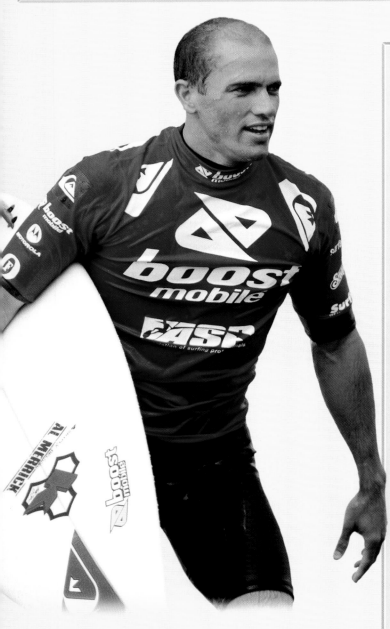

Kelly Slater has been called the Michael Jordan of surfing. Slater currently holds more surfing championship titles than anyone else in the world.

Surfing has changed a great deal since Captain Cook arrived in Hawaii. Ever since surfing had its renaissance, or "new beginning," in the 1960s, it has become a sport that has attracted much attention from advertisers and sponsors worldwide. By the late 1970s, surfing contests had begun popping up all over the world. They were not only in Hawaii, California, and Australia, but in South Africa, Japan, and Brazil. Large international sponsors like Coca-Cola are willing to give huge money prizes to the best of the best in the ocean. For those who have risen to the top, surfing can be a very lucrative pastime.

Pro Surfing

In 1977, surfing promoter Fred Hemmings Jr., organized a worldwide surf tour for professionals. It took place in thirteen separate contests across the globe. The tour was a resounding success and pro surfing was here to stay.

Although the contests helped the sport become an international pastime with coverage on radio and television, there were flaws in the system. Thanks to changing wave conditions, surfers in competitions sometimes had completely different surf experiences. Different waves allowed different maneuvers, which affected points and scoring. One surfer might be lucky enough to catch the perfect wave, while another equally talented surfer might never catch a decent wave. Since the contests were judged mainly on these maneuvers, this caused a dilemma in scoring.

Another problem with such contests was how one entered the competition. Getting into a competition was nearly impossible unless you knew someone important such as another pro surfer or a competition judge. A fair way to enter surfers' competitions became extremely important for contest organizers. Because surfing is traditionally such an exclusive sport (getting onto any great surf spot is very difficult for the newcomer), it was difficult for rookies to break into the pro circuit.

To solve this problem, events like the Pro Class Trials were created. In these events, unknown surfers from across the globe have a fair chance at entering the contests. Today there are several huge surfing competitions that use trials to admit new, unknown surfers. These competitions occur worldwide throughout the year. After all, just because it's winter in North America doesn't mean the waves aren't hot in Australia.

Scoring a Surf Competition

In terms of scoring a surfing competition, the criteria have changed significantly over the years. Traditionally, one whole ride was scored by a judge. Now, each special move or maneuver is judged with a specific amount of points awarded. The surfer receives points during his or her allotted time in the waves (often fifteen minutes in length), which are added together for his or her score.

Usually, the competitions are arranged in heats, or short trials in which the surfers have a chance to prove their stuff. These heats can last anywhere from five minutes to fifteen minutes, sometimes even longer. In some heats, four surfers compete at the same time. Most competitions have both individual and team events.

All competitions have slightly different rules, but for the most part, competition scoring has four parts: Radically Controlled Maneuvers, Most Critical Section, the Biggest and/or Best Waves, and Longest Functional Distance. These criteria are decided by the International Surfing Association (ISA), the organization that oversees most contests worldwide. Scoring and rules may vary in different regions and in competitions run by smaller organizations.

The Endless Summer

In 1966, when California was buzzing about surfing, filmmaker/surfer Bruce Brown made the classic documentary *The Endless Summer*. The film charted the adventures of surfers Robert August and Mike Hynson as they searched the globe for "the perfect wave." Their travels led them to places where few, if any, had surfed before—Africa, Australia, and even parts of South America. The movie was a huge hit, especially among the surfing culture. In 2002, Brown's son Dana made another surfing movie, *Step into Liquid*, in his father's tradition. Thanks to the Browns and other surfing filmmakers, we have unique footage to view when learning about and appreciating this amazing sport.

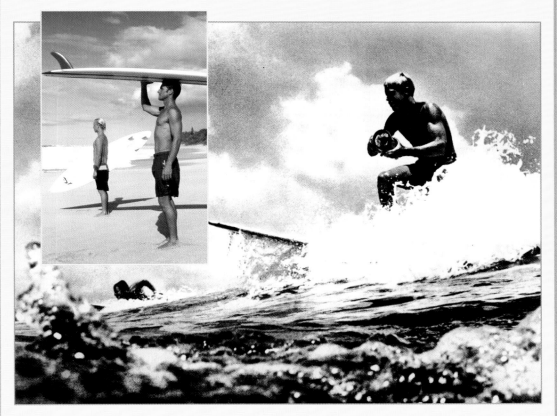

After seeing the documentary *The Endless Summer,* many Californians left their home beaches and went on their own search for the perfect wave. Here, filmmaker Bruce Brown rides a wave while capturing action on film for his movie.

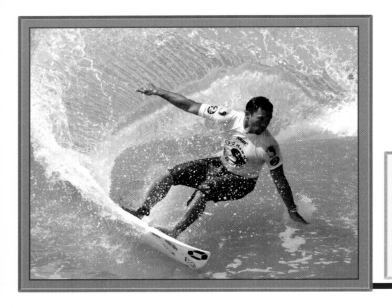

Sunny Garcia discovered surfing when he was thrown into the ocean by his prankster friends. Then only seven years old, Garcia rode the waves back to the shore. Today, he is considered one of the best surfers in the world.

Today's Surfing Superstars

Many surfing superstars have come and gone. Today, three surfers are acknowledged as the active legends of the sport—Kelly Slater, Sunny Garcia, and Rob Machado.

One of the world's most talented surfers, Kelly Slater has competed in the Association of Surfing Professionals circuit for more than ten years. He has won six world championships, a world record in itself.

Slater has graced the cover of many surfing magazines and has a full line of endorsements. Some call him the best surfer of all time. Aside from the near million dollars he has earned in contest money, he has brought home more than twice that amount in endorsements. These accomplishments, along with the skill and determination required to be the best athlete in any sport, make him an international surfing superstar.

Sunny Garcia has remained on the list of international surfing's top sixteen players for a decade. Garcia is one of the most recognizable surfing stars. He has been competing on the international circuit for more than seventeen years and has earned in excess of $900,000 in winnings in his career.

Rob Machado is one of the most famous goofyfoot surfers of all time. At he age of 11, Machado began surfing while living in San Diego, California. He remains in the top league of surfers and has mastered almost every major contest there is.

Women in Surfing

Even in ancient Hawaii, women and men surfed the waves side by side. Since surfing regained popularity in the twentieth century, women have participated in the sport as well. In fact, when Duke Paoa Kahanamoku visited Australia with his surfboard in 1915, a woman rode with him. Her name was Isabel Letham, and she was the first Australian ever to surf!

Like women in politics, business, and other professions have struggled to receive recognition for their achievements, so have women in the world of surfing. The pioneers of women's surfing provided the inspiration for the younger generations of women to come. Television and the movies also played a role in opening the door for women surfers. During the 1960s, Gidget was a popular character in several movies and a television series. Gidget was a young girl who spent her summers surfing in Malibu, California. The popularity of this character inspired many young women to try surfing. Soon enough, there were many women joining the lineup, riding the waves right alongside the men.

Surfing girls sometimes have a different mentality than their male counterparts. Female surfing pioneers Rella Sunn and Jericho Poppler from Hawaii commented in *The History of Surfing*: "Boys are out there to prove they can conquer the waves . . . but girls are more like artists who work their choreography and go out to dance routines set up by the situation the waves dictate."

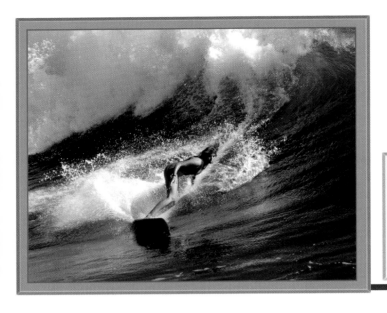

Despite her parents' wishes, Lisa Anderson persisted in becoming a professional surfer. During the late 1980s, she honed her skills in the California surf.

In the 1960s, the most respected and recognizable woman surfer was Margo Godfrey. She competed well into the 1970s and won the Bells Beach women's division in Australia. Following Godfrey's lead, in the 1980s Pam Burridge dazzled the surfing world with her talented boardwork. Since the 1990s, another surfer, named Lisa Anderson, has emerged as a star and has collected thirty-five trophies in the contest circuit. Anderson remains a role model for aspiring women surfers. And their love for surfing has never stopped. In 1997, seven pioneers of women's surfing posed for a portrait. Even though several are now white-haired grandmothers, they still admit to surfing all the time!

Modern Technology and Surfing

For those aspiring surfers who live near the coastline, there are always plenty of waves. Seaside towns, especially those known for having great surfing spots, are perfect places for kids to get a year-round education in surfing. But for kids who are landlocked, living nowhere near the ocean, there are alternatives.

Wave Pools

Wave pools give people all over the world, regardless of their geographic location, the opportunity to try surfing. Through the use of high-powered pumps and reservoirs, wave pools simulate the ocean. The machinery in wave pools has evolved so that today they incorporate all different types of waves into their repertoire, including halfpipes and easy peaks.

Tow-Ins

Tow-ins began in the 1970s. Surfers had always known that the biggest waves sometimes crash miles from the coast on outer reefs— far out of reach from the paddling surfer. In the twentieth century, the creation of wave vehicles like jet skis made reaching the biggest waves possible. Large boats and even helicopters are sometimes used to assist the surfer in making it to the outer reefs.

After being towed in, the surfer generally uses a special board— one fitted with straps fastened to the board to keep the surfer safely atop and attached securely to the board. Although some surfers use smaller boards (seven feet two and up), the bulk of tow-in surfers prefer the big guns (nine feet six and up), mainly because of the power they give the surfer. Tow-in surfing is extremely dangerous, and only surfing daredevils will even attempt it. They describe the experience as completely unique—something they will do for the rest of their lives.

Spin-Off Sports

Since the popularity of surfing exploded in the 1960s, manufacturers have tried to devise spin-off surfing activities. This expanded the market and really targeted some surfers' needs.

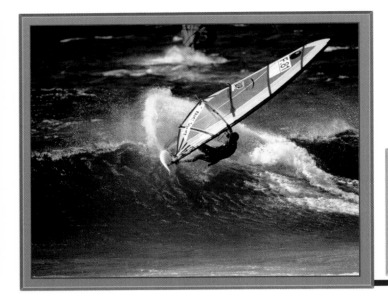

Windsurfing can be quite an acrobatic sport. Many windsurfers perform amazing stunts that involve twists, turns, and leaps into the air.

Skateboarding

Surfing's most popular spin-off is undoubtedly skateboarding. Introduced in 1963, skateboarding became a national craze almost overnight. Before long, however, kids started losing interest, and by the mid-1960s, the skateboard had all but disappeared.

Then a team of bad-boy surfers from an area of a Southern California beach nicknamed "Dogtown" turned to skateboarding after the precious morning waves had subsided for the day. During surfing downtime, these kids—called the Zephyr Skate Team—practiced their surfing moves on skateboards day in and day out. When they saw famous surfer Larry Bertlemann do a cutback for the first time, they decided to attempt it on a skateboard. Thus, modern-day skateboarding was born all because a few bored surfers couldn't catch their waves!

Windsurfing

In the 1930s, surfer Tom Blake began toying with attaching sails to his surfboard. It wasn't until the 1980s, however, that windsurfing became a popular sport. The benefits of surfing with a sail were obvious: no paddling, few crowds, and very high speeds. The windsurfer can also ride all different kinds of waves. Since the surfer is propelled by the force of the wind, windsurfing requires much less effort on the part of the surfer.

Snowboarding

Snowboarding is the perfect marriage of surfing and skiing. Instead of wearing two skis, the participant is firmly strapped to a surfboardlike board. With this innovation, it is possible to surf mountaintops covered in snow! In other words, the snowboard basically surfs waves of snow. The sport has really taken off over the past decade, and ski resorts have even included halfpipes on their slopes for hotdogging snowboarders.

Go Catch a Wave!

There are lots of ways to get started and learn about surfing, even if you don't live near a beach! There are numerous Web sites where you can learn about contests and surfing celebrities, surfing equipment, competition rules, and so on. There are even chat rooms for young surfers like yourself, just wanting to learn more about the sport.

The Hawaiians knew it, and now the world does, too—there's nothing like surfing! As this ancient pastime has stepped into its new identity as a contemporary craze, the world cannot get enough of surfing. Not only is it fun, but talented surfers can even make careers out of their favorite pastime.

One of the things that will keep the wannabe surfer coming back for more is the simplicity of the sport. With just a body and a board, surfers have discovered that it is possible to become one with nature, simply by riding its billowing waves, having fun, and being stoked.

Time shows that surfing is here to stay. With the arrival of new surf stars on the contest circuit, it is obvious that this trend will continue for years to come.

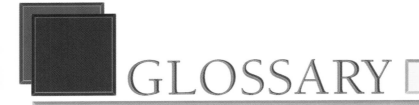

GLOSSARY

buoyant   Having the ability to float.

bypass   To pass by going around.

cumbersome   Difficult to handle because of weight or bulk.

evoke   To call forth or bring out.

fiberglass   A material made of glass and plastics.

heat   A round in a race or competition.

instinctive   Done on impulse; spontaneous and unthinking.

lingo   The special language of a particular field of interest.

lucrative   Producing wealth.

maneuver   An intended and controlled movement.

missionary   A person sent to a foreign country to carry on an activity, especially religious.

novice   A person new to a field or activity; a beginner.

reservoirs   Bodies of stored water.

FOR MORE INFORMATION

Eastern Surfing Association
P.O. Box 582
Ocean City, MD 21843
(866) SURF-ESA (787-3372)
Web site: http://www.surfesa.org/home

International Surfing Association
5580 La Jolla Blvd. PMB 145
La Jolla, CA 92037
(858) 551-5292

International Surfing Museum
P.O. Box 782
Huntington Beach, CA 92648
Web site: http://www.surfingmuseum.org

Web Sites

Due to the changing nature of Internet links, the Rosen Publishing Group, Inc., has developed an online list of Web sites related to the subject of this book. This site is updated regularly. Please use this link to access the list:

http//:www.rosenlinks.com/scc/surf

FOR FURTHER READING

Bass, Scott. *Surf! Your Guide to Longboarding, Shortboarding, Tubing, Aerials, Hanging Ten and More.* Washington, DC: National Geographic, 2003.

Dixon, Peter. *The Complete Guide to Surfing.* Guilford, CT: Lyons Press, 2004.

Fredaini, Paul. *Surf Flex: Flexibility, Yoga, and Conditioning Exercises for Surfers.* Long Island City, NY: Hatherleigh Press, 2001.

Kampion, Drew. *Stoked! A History of Surf Culture.* Layton, VT: Gibbs Smith, 2003.

Slater, Kelly, with Jason Barte. *Pipe Dreams: A Surfer's Journey.* New York: Regan Books, 2004.

Warshaw, Matt. *The Encyclopedia of Surfing.* New York: Harcourt, 2003.

Werner, Doug. *Longboarder's Start-Up: A Guide to Longboard Surfing* (Start-Up Sports Series, No. 6). Chula Vista, CA: Tracks Publishing, 1996.

Werner, Doug. *Surfer's Start-Up: A Beginner's Guide to Surfing.* Chula Vista, CA: Tracks Publishing, 1999.

Zakarin, Debra Mostow. *Surf's Up!: A Surf Style Handbook.* New York: Grosset & Dunlap, 2002.

BIBLIOGRAPHY

Bizley, Kirk. *Surfing*. Chicago: Heinemann Library Press, 2000.

Cralle, Trevor. *The Surfin'ary: A Dictionary of Surfing Terms and Surf Speak*. Berkeley, CA: Ten Speed Press, 2001.

Hemmings, Fred. *The Soul of Surfing*. New York: Thunder's Mouth Press, 1997.

Maclaren, James. *Learn to Surf*. New York: Lyons and Burford, 1997.

Turner, Stephen. *Windsurfing*. New York: Gallery Books, 1986.

Young, Nat, with Craig McGregor. *The History of Surfing*. Tucson, AZ: Body Press, 1987.

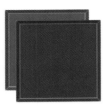

INDEX

A
accessories, 15–19, 21
Anderson, Lisa, 38
Anderson, Simon, 15
Association of Surfing
    Professionals, 36
August, Robert, 35

B
Bells Beach Contest, 15, 38
Bertlemann, Larry, 40
Blake, Tom, 40
boogie boards, 18
Brown, Bruce, 35
Brown, Dana, 35
Burridge, Pam, 38

C
competitions
   entering, 33–34
   scoring in, 34
Cook, Captain James, 4–5, 9, 10, 32
custom boards, 14

D
dropping in, 29
duckdiving, 22
Duke, the (Duke Paoa Kahanamoku),
    8, 37
Duke Classic, the, 8

E
Endless Summer, The, 35
etiquette, 26–31

F
fiberglass boards, 10, 11, 14
fins, 14–15, 22

G
Garcia, Sunny, 36
Godfrey, Margo, 38

H
Hawaii, 4–5, 6–9, 11, 12, 18, 32,
    37, 41
helping others, 26–27
Hemmings, Fred, Jr., 33
History of Surfing, The, 37
hostility, avoiding, 27
Hui Nalu Club, 8
Hynson, Mike, 35

I
International Surfing Association, 34

L
leash, 12, 16–17, 21
Letham, Isabel, 27
lineup, 22–24, 26, 27, 29, 30, 31, 37

lingo, 31
longboards, 11–12, 13, 31

M
Machado, Rob, 36, 37
molded boards, 14

N
noseguards, 17–19

O
Oahu, Hawaii, 12, 18

P
Poppler, Jericho, 37
popup, 20–21, 24
Pro Class Trials, 34
pro surfing, 33–34

R
right of way, 26
riptides, 30–31

S
safety, 29
sharks, 28
shortboards, 13
skateboarding, 40

skim boards, 18
Slater, Kelly, 36
snowboarding, 41
soft boards, 12, 14
sponsors/endorsements,
    32, 36
Step into Liquid, 35
Sunn, Rella, 37
sunscreen, 30
surfboards
    evolution of, 10–12, 15
    holding on to, 27
surfboard shapers, 11, 14
surfing
    history of, 4–9
    learning, 20–26
    today, 32–41

T
tow-ins, 39

W
wave, catching, 24–26
wave pools, 39
wax, 15–16
wet suits, 19
white water, 22
windsurfing, 40–41
women surfers, 37–38

About the Author

When she is not traveling the globe competing in surfing competitions, Naima Green works as a freelance writer in New York City.

Photo Credits

Cover, pp. 1, 3, 5, 11, 14, 15, 16, 17, 18, 19, 20, 21, 23, 25, 27, 29, 30, 33 Robert Hudson/The Rosen Publishing Group; p. 4 © Hulton-Deutsch Collection/Corbis; p. 7 Collection Kharbine-Tapabor, Paris, France/www.bridgeman.co.uk; pp. 8, 10 © Bettman/Corbis; pp. 13, 38, 40 © Rick Doyle/Corbis; p. 28 © Kurt Jones/Icon SMI; p. 32 © Stan Liu/Icon SMI; p. 35 © Hulton/Archive/Getty Images; p. 35 (inset) © Howard Jacqueline/Corbis Sygma; p. 36 © Reuters/Corbis.

Thanks to Newport Harbor High School, Newport Beach, California, and to Surfside Sports, Newport Beach, California

Designer: Nelson Sá; **Editor:** Charles Hofer;
Photo Researcher: Adriana Skura